Moving Your Patients to YES!

Easy Insurance Conversations

Teresa Duncan, M.S.

Moving Your Patients to YES!

Printed by:
CreateSpace Independent Publishing Platform

Copyright © 2017, Odyssey Management, Inc.

Published in the United States of America

Book ID: 160503-00411

ISBN-13: 978-1548222505
ISBN-10: 154822250X

Here's What's Inside...

Introduction

Moving Your Patients to Yes!

I have been in the dental field for over 20 years and have worked in each and every (unlicensed) position in the office. I know the pressure to be the person who must move a patient to 'yes' in the middle of a busy day. It took me years of practice and learning what works to perfect what I share with you in this book.

Dental insurance will become a bigger part of dental offices as the future unfolds. If we don't acknowledge its effect and find a way to have effective conversations, then we will find ourselves behind the curve. You may be competing with offices that will be good at these conversations and the patients will feel much more confident visiting them to have procedures done. I want *you* to have the verbal skills to make your insurance conversations easy so you can move your patients to 'yes.'

I see the hesitation in the faces of people who attend my classes. A frequent question is "How do I get this patient to say 'yes'? How do I get the patient to accept treatment?" Use what you learn from the book to form a better bond with the patient so that they not only hear you but *listen to you.*

I hope this book helps your team to discuss those sticky financial options with your patients. My goal is to inspire your team to enter your patient conversations with confidence and the knowledge that your recommendations are for the patient's benefit.

Here's To Your Success!

Teresa Duncan, M.S.

How Can Dental Insurance Coordinators Move Their Clients to 'Yes'?

The challenge for dental insurance coordinators is that so much information must be given to a patient within a small amount of time. By the time we are in front of the patient, they are already tired from their appointment and they want nothing more than to get out of the office. They have had an emotional conversation with the doctor and found out they need a lot of treatment. By the time the insurance coordinator is able to review with them their benefits and finances, the patients' minds are often racing and they feel overwhelmed. It's a very unique skill set to be able to effectively 'speak' both clinically and financially with a patient. Typically, those are two different skill sets in the office and it is hard to find someone who is comfortable with money matters *and* who can also talk bone height and grafts.

I often hear from team members who wish they had more training in the softer skill of conversation. They're under a lot of pressure to learn the software skills; how the practice files claims; and the onerous HIPAA and OSHA requirements. But true practice success comes from the soft side – how you interact with your patients and how they respond to your treatment recommendations.

Most dental professionals have not received this training in their dental schools or programs.The focus is usually on clinial and time management skills, not people skills. Hopefully you can find employees who have this innate 'gift' to talk easily with patients. Most offices however will have to train team members regularly to keep up with patient concerns. Hopefully, this book will help with the training process.

With a little practice and some coaching, most of our client's team members are able to successfully have these conversations. They often just need to have the pathway laid out for them. Once they find their groove, they'll be able to do this with their eyes closed. They'll know exactly what to say and when to say it in order to move the patient to 'yes!

Don't Focus on their Insurance - Focus on Their Oral Health

Patients will always have questions about money and affordability. There's no getting away from it. Patients don't typically announce, "Yes, just do whatever you'd like and I'll pay for it." By assuming that patients will have questions we can prepare for those conversations. To be an effective dental team, we need to be able to serve the patients - not just clinically, but also financially. When we are able to show the patient that we know what we're talking about as far as their benefits, eligibility and co-payment amounts, they will begin to trust us. Why? Because they'll know we have their best interests at heart.

"We want to heal you AND we want to help you afford your treatment."

The fee matters. Whether you're counting dollars or pennies – it's consumer behavior to want to know the price paid for a service. By recognizing and tackling one of the patients' biggest concerns to moving forward with treatment - the fact that they often can't afford it - we can show our patients our role as a resource, not an obstacle. It means offices who can build this trust will be busier; and *that* means increased oral health for our patients.

It is helpful to have more than one person in the office who knows how to answer these questions. Every team member should have the conversations in this book practiced and prepared so they can handle any questions coming at them. These questions come to us on the phone, in the operatory and sometimes in passing out business cards in public. We can't rely on just one or two key people who can answer all the questions. A team that is on board with the practice's philosophy should be able to ease patient fears anywhere, anytime.

Our patients would like to use their dental benefits, but often don't understand the plan provisions. Dental insurance coordinators, act as a translator between the dental plan and getting the treatment done. If we can help the patient utilize their plan in the best manner, then the patient will be thrilled. Look at it from their point of view: they have a product they're paying for but they don't quite understand what they're receiving. This confusion leads to unclear expectations.

We're the ones with the secret. We understand how to read this strange language in a dental contract. The offices that are able to provide this valuable translation service will find their patients trust they have their best interests at heart.

We're able to help them improve their oral health by learning these verbal skills that help us have these informative conversations with our patients. We know patients who put off dental treatment end up with more expensive and more painful dental treatment. If we're able to help them have treatment sooner, then they can avoid the possibility of a lifelong struggle with pain and infection.

You have examples in your own offices of patients who put off treatment. Try to think of these situations to put together a graphic or cheat sheet of the cost involved. Use the example below but populate with your own fees. These are examples only.

Situation: Patient opts for a three-unit anterior bridge. Three years later, an obvious bony defect appears.

Treatment - Round 1:
Total cost of bridge with buildups $ 3,750

Treatment - Round 2:
Cost of corrective treatment three years later:

Bone graft	**$ 1,000**
Implant/abutment/crown	**$ 5,000**
2 crowns (without endo)	**$ 2,200**
Total Cost	**$11,950**

Refer to the appendix for more examples.

By showing our patients that postponing treatment is in fact detrimental to their financial health as well as oral health, our argument becomes more persuasive. The numbers above are hard to contest. Patients don't have the experience we do in knowing the longevity of procedures. With visuals and calculations like the one above, your position will be better supported.

In the end, we are here to improve the lives of our patients. We know firsthand the difference that poor oral health can make for a person. Keep this in mind, when you find yourself wanting to rush a conversation or are just going through the motions. **Our patients will not receive a better answer to their dental questions than from us**. The procedures performed in your office can be life-changing. Never forget that.

Words Matter

<u>Oops!</u>

In conversations with patients, what you say makes a difference! Often, you will hear you shouldn't say "Oops," or "I don't know" to a patient and it is absolutely true! We don't want to say "oops" because we don't want the patient to think a procedure has gone wrong. Imagine if you were in the chair and you heard "uh-oh" behind you – you would be scared! Our confidence has to shine through at all times. If you encounter an issue in the operatory then it's best to tap the clinician on the arm to convey that you need to stop. That's an easy fix – don't say "oops!" But what about the other common jargon that may fly under the radar? Let's give each other permission to eavesdrop on one another.

Constructive criticism is an essential trait of a highly successful team. If you listen to each other as a team then you'll hear snippets of conversation that you could probably tweak. This is natural and helpful. I would ask you to listen to your team members and make note if semi-professional or 'easy' terms are being used. Dentists and team members tend to not want to upset patients and as a result, we soften our message. Is this happening in your office?

Just A Cleaning

We tend to say "just a cleaning" when we mean
"**hygiene appointment**" or "**preventive
therapy**." Your hygienists will give you guidance
on what you should call it. "Just a cleaning" is not
accurate and minimizes the impact of the
services we provide. When patients call to
change their appointments often they'll
apologize for having to do it. Are you (out of
habit) responding with "Well, don't worry. It's
just a cleaning"? This phrase undermines the
important work that we do. Listen to the phone
calls around you. Typically, this happens simply
because no one has pointed it out. The good
news is that it is an easy correction.

Cancellations

Another frequently used term is 'cancellation.'
Let's try to avoid this word. Instead, use the
phrase "**change in the schedule**." If the patient
calls to cancel then respond with, "I'm sorry we
have to **change the schedule.** I'd like to
schedule you for (soonest opening)." Be
assumptive in your rescheduling!

Another reason to not use "cancellation" is
patient perception. We don't want the patient to
think this is a normal occurrence in the office.
When you say "it's okay if you cancel – we'll just

fill it" then that absolutely sends the wrong message to the patient. We want the patient to know how sorry we are about the change and that it's important to us to reschedule the appointment as soon as possible.

Insurance Talk

What are the softened messages in insurance? They're not so much softened as they are inaccurate. Our insurance language revolves around contract clauses and limitations. As a result, we speak in "legal-ese" when discussing insurance. Let's review some of the terms often used. As dental insurance coordinators, we tend to say "maximum" when talking with patients about their benefit breakdowns. Start calling it a "**yearly benefit**" instead. A maximum means that they can only use a certain amount of money.

It also implies a stopping point. When a patient reaches their "maximum" then they may think they have to stop with dental treatment. I remember a patient who would only proceed with one crown per year. When I asked him if he'd consider continuing with his treatment he told me that he would be happy to. I was shocked! I asked him why he didn't say anything at his last appointment and he told me "well, I thought we had to stick to the maximum." He simply didn't understand that he could proceed with treatment but just pay for it out of pocket. It was an eye-opener for me. I realized that some people take words at face value.

Remember that dental insurance isn't like traditional medical, home or auto insurance. There is no large payout for necessary care. Instead, patients are given an amount of money per year. For this reason, I'd like you to call it a "**yearly benefit**." Once this benefit is paid out to the patient then the insurance plan is all but forgotten until the next benefit year.

When a patient hears that a procedure is "not covered" their first thought is to not move forward. They've been conditioned with medical and traditional home insurance non-coverage deterring any action. By removing "not covered" from our conversations then we are not planting subconscious stopping points. Let's look at it from the patient's point of view: it's easy for them to come to the conclusion that it's not important enough to be covered.

On the medical side, many procedures aren't covered or are severely scrutinized. Unfortunately, on the medical side, when patients hear that procedures aren't covered, they tend to opt out. We see the same behavior in dentistry.

What we are trying to convey is that benefits don't exist for their procedure *but* we can still make it affordable. An alternate way of discussing non-coverage is "your insurance company isn't going to provide a benefit for that service. Let's talk about how we can help." The patient is hearing an explanation and an offer of help rather than simply "it's not covered."

It is important to listen to our words and the words our team members are using. As a team, listen and evaluate if your conversations are filled with words which minimize our impact on the patient.

What to Stop Saying to Your Patients

I hear some very strange and interesting conversations when I visit offices and listen to recorded calls. Owners and managers should strongly consider a call recording system to evaluate the effectiveness of your patient conversations. Many training opportunities can be identified by taking five to ten minutes of your day to listen in on key phone calls. Start by listening to the longest calls and the new patient calls. As a manager, this is highly valuable information. Call monitoring systems are widely available and may already be a part of your existing phone or patient reminder system. Check with your dental society to make sure call recording is legal in your state.

As a result of observing many offices and listening in on countless phone conversations, I'm going to give you some of the top conversation busters I've heard.

Criticizing their insurance. We don't want to point out how bad their plan is. I have heard receptionists say, "**We see a lot of plans like yours**. You know, a lot of them are not that great. **Yours is definitely one of the worst**." Don't be the one who breaks this news to your patient! I have also heard, "**Your plan barely covers anything. Honestly - your plan isn't that great**."

Keep in mind that patients aren't usually responsible for choosing their dental plan. When we point out bad aspects of their plan, it's not serving any good purpose except to make them upset and even more confused. Many of them assumed they had decent benefits. If they are not familiar with insurance plans, then why would they think differently? This news is discouraging for them to hear. Instead of pointing out how bad someone's plan is, let's use this information as a way to comfort the patient by helping them *figure out* their benefits. With this tactic, we can then help them decide which treatment they would like to pursue and how we can make it affordable.

Check your own benefits. Time and again, I hear from team members who are too overwhelmed and busy to properly obtain benefit verification. Often they'll take the chance that the benefits will be simple to explain. Unfortunately, with these plans usually come the weirdest clauses. The office that depends on the patient to know their benefits will find themselves writing off amounts due to angry patients.

If your message to your patient is "**Check your benefits and get back to me**," then you are really saying to the patient: "I'm too busy for you right now. You handle your benefits, and come back to us when you're ready." I'm sure you know this will not happen. When a patient decides to call the office, they have made a huge decision to move forward with scheduling. If they hear that we're not going to help them with their benefits, then can you blame them for wanting to find a different office? I don't.

Busy offices tend to be guilty of this and it is usually a matter of priority. The thought could be that the patient in the office is more important than the potential appointment. In reality, all patients should be valued. If a patient hears "I'm not sure what your benefits are, so go ahead and look into it, and give me a call back," you can bet the patient will not call back. This happens more than most dental offices would care to admit, unfortunately. With call recording spot-checks, you can quickly identify if this is happening in your office.

Come back with new insurance. Imagine calling an office after checking the insurance website to find a convenient provider. You look up the provider's website to confirm that they take your plan. When you call the office to make an appointment the office lets you know that not only did they cease participation but they are rude once they hear your plan's name. I have heard dental team members say, "**We'll never work with your plan again, so if you switch to another one, let us know**." That's writing off the patient's value to the office. You've effectively shut them down.

Your bad experience with a plan should have absolutely no bearing on the care that we provide to our patients. Many patients will have a plan that you won't like. Actually – most patients will have plans you won't like. I urge you not to bring your bias into the conversation. My favorite statement was: "**Oh, you have *THAT* plan**."

I don't think I need to explain why this is such a bad statement! It was condescending and resulted in the patient telling the receptionist that she needed a lesson in manners. And the patient was right.

Verbal Foundations for Your Team

When starting off with a new mindset it's helpful to have foundational terms to give it voice. Go-to terms help when you're feeling flustered, lose control of the conversation or if you receive unexpected questions. I recommend writing these down on a sticky note and keeping it nearby. In this electronic age, why a sticky note? If you need to refer to it quickly, you can pull it out of your lab coat pocket, refer to your computer monitor or look at the note in the break room. Patients are great at throwing us for a loop – even the most experienced team member can become flustered!

My favorite go-to comments are meant to re-assure the patient that they are not an unusual case. Patients are already self-conscious about needed treatment. Remember they may have not seen a dentist for years and are embarrassed. How we respond will impact their decision to stay with us for treatment or if they will continue to put it off.

"We have a lot of patients who ..." This statement helps the patient to feel comfortable with our experience. The message is that we've dealt with their plan; their situation; or similar concerns and we are here to help.   Your patient doesn't want to feel that this is the first time you've had an issue. It increases their level of nervousness. By making a 'soothing' comment such as "other patients with your plan have found that..." we can allay their fears enough to find out what else is concerning to them. Other examples of when to use this term:

- We have several patients who are able to submit to a health savings account.
- We've helped many patients use their benefits.
- We've been able to help patients decide between benefits or our dental savings club.

"**We have found that** ..." This is also an effective phrase to use - especially when discussing a patient's coverage for specific treatment. Patients are naturally curious as to how much the plan will pay and look to us for this information. This is why it's important for us to be confident with our information.

- "We have found that with patients on this particular plan, we seem to have more difficulty getting reimbursement for this procedure."
- "We have found that this plan pays at 80%, but the reimbursement is closer to 70%."
- "We have found that appealing procedures with this plan is more difficult than expected."

Basically, we're saying we have familiarity with *that* particular plan. "**Many of our patients have your insurance - we do have experience with your plan**." This is what a new patient wants to hear. What you're doing with that sentence is reinforcing that they made the right decision; that they are coming to the right office; and that you *will* take care of them.

One of my favorite phrases is, "**We can check into your plan for you**." This is a reflection of a team that understands customer service will bring them back every time. Instead of saying to a patient, "I'm not sure what your benefits are going to cover," or, "Go ahead and look into it, and let us know what you find out," we are taking on their burden. It's a promise to the patient and when we follow through it builds trust.

Once we obtain their information and check into the plan for them then we've communicated our capability and our caring. I love being the one who offers this service to the patient. I have no doubt that when the patient calls another office, they will not receive the same level of service. Team members who are customer-service oriented will enjoy this part of their task as it allows them to communicate in a very positive way with an uncertain patient.

'Premier' and 'Preferred'? What Do You Mean

Handling inquiries for Delta Dental plans can become very confusing which leads to a frustrated mindset. As you know, insurance companies have different tiers and different networks. It's common for a patient to come in with the belief that they are part of one network, and unfortunately, they're part of a different network - a lower paying network. I'm going to give you some verbal skills for dealing with a patient who isn't aware of the two different levels and is not sure how to handle the difference in the benefits. What is your response when a patient says, "What do you mean, 'premier'? What are you talking about?"

Your goal with this conversation is to convey that yes, there are different levels and the reimbursement will be different. However, it doesn't mean the patient cannot come to your office. It means there is a difference in reimbursement level.

"I'm not sure if you knew that Delta offered two levels, but there's a Preferred and a Premier level. If you could share your information, I can find out your benefits, check into it and get back to you in the next 24 hours."

Patients will ask why your office is a member of one network and not a member of another. What's tricky about this explanation is that you are saying the office will not be paid as much. It's a real-world situation but it can sound wrong if it's not delivered well.

- "We took a good look at both plans, and it just didn't work out for us to be a member of the preferred level. We decided to stay a member of the premier level."
- "We crunched the numbers, and it just wasn't working for us, and so this is why we belong to this network instead."

After clarifying to which network you belong, the patient is left wondering, "What does this mean for me?" It is now our job to convey that the patient could (and should!) still come to your office. The challenge is that the copayment amounts will be different. Not necessarily prohibitive but different. Practice these lines with your team:

- "The good news is you can still come here! Nothing changes with your claims, Mrs. Smith. We'll still submit your claims for you."
- "The good news is we're going to check your benefits for you to find out the difference. Then I'll let you know."

- "The good news is we will do the work for you on our end."

Nothing is more terrifying than telling a patient they will have to file their own claim!

Even if you are not dealing with Delta Dental plans you may have plans with different benefit tiers. Within one insurance company there can be a large number of plans – all of them different from each other. It's imperative to have the proper benefit information so you can provide the most accurate information.

Your administrative team should be able to explain the difference between Delta's Premier and Preferred plans. If the clinical team is aware then that's great but at a minimum, the team answering the phones must know this. After dealing with different benefit tiers you'll be able to confidently discuss them. This comes from multiple times researching and discussing the tiers. Ideally we'd like you to be able to make explanations like the ones below – with clarity and confidence!

- "We are familiar with your plan, and we can tell you that it's going to work this way."
- "We have checked your plan and it seems crowns are paid at a lower percentage."

What happens if you're not sure? That's okay! Ask the patient for a little time to research the issue. The important piece is to follow up. Lack of follow up erodes the trust patients are slow to build. It's perfectly fine to ask for 24 hours to look into the matter. A simple "I'd like to check your benefits, and I'll call you back by this time tomorrow" works just fine!

"Why Don't You Participate With My Insurance?"

Sometimes a patient will not understand why you've chosen to move out of network or are not listed on their plan's site. When a patient asks you about this, be <u>sympathetic and positive</u>. Why is that underlined? Because our inner voice is listing many reasons but none the patient wants to hear. What the patient is really asking is 'what does this mean for me?'

Your response should be "**We *do* take your insurance**." Most offices will file a claim and help with deciphering benefits. A deeper answer is that you've reviewed the two plans and found they don't work for your office. It's fair to inform the patient of this. Honestly, your patient will not be surprised. The climate of insurance today is that consumers realize physicians and dentists aren't paid very much. The news that you've performed your due diligence won't really surprise anyone. Here are some gentle ways to break the information:

- "The doctor reviewed the plan and found the amount of reimbursement wouldn't cover the cost of providing your care."
- "But we will work with your insurance. We will be happy to file the claim for you. What I can do is find out how your plan will work in our office. I don't want you to have any surprises when you come to our office, and I know you don't want any surprises, either."

If you've crunched the numbers and found the fee schedule was not fair, I have absolutely no issue with you sharing this information with the patient. That last paragraph is important in reassuring the patient. We really don't want our patients to have surprises. Your patients will most likely not be aware of the differences between in- and out-of-network providers. Make sure you are aware of the differences and that your team understands how claims are processed.

The difference between participation and non-participation is:

- You don't have to accept their fee schedule if you don't participate.

- The payment may not come to you – even if you are assigned the benefits. Many plans will not pay out-of-network providers.
- The benefit levels may differ slightly or wildly.

If you are aware that a plan always sends the check to the patient, then you should notify the patient of this fact upfront. They will need to cover the cost of the visit but you will file their claim for them.

Patients will often say, "Well, why can't you just have the check come to you?" This is the unfortunate truth and you'll need to deliver it in a nice manner:

"We know your plan will not send us the benefits. We have many patients with this plan and they will cover the visit. Don't worry – we'll file the claim with any necessary paperwork and you'll receive the check directly from them."

It's unfortunate that many patients are not able to pay their health care bills without a payment plan. For this reason, a financial presentation helps them to plan ahead for treatment. Third party financing such as CareCredit can help them afford the care they need.

If the check is unexpectedly sent to the patient, you'll need to call them to explain why.
And to attempt collection of the benefits! You could kindly explain that the check should have come to you and combine this with the assumption they will make payment.

"We talked with your insurance company today and they said they sent payment to you. Next time you are in we can make sure to take that into account. While I have you on the phone, I can take your credit card number and settle up your account with us."

Or if they are not willing to give you payment information:

"We talked with your insurance company today and they said they sent payment to you. Next time you are in we can make sure to take that into account. What I'll do is send you a payment link/statement via email and you can handle it when you are home. If you change your mind and want to give me a credit card, just let me know."

Being an out-of-network provider doesn't mean you're an out-of-luck provider! It simply means you'll have to be very clear about payment expectations and how payments work in your office. Patients do expect to pay for care but it's up to you set the expectation that co-payments are meant to be collected!

<u>"Why Don't You Know My Benefits?"</u>

This question is great, isn't it? We deal with so many patients every day with a great variety of plans. Some of you are dealing with hundreds if not thousands of plans in your databases. Patients are famous for arriving at our offices and assuming that we know the ins and outs of every dental plan in our database. I'm always impressed by the very sharp insurance coordinators who do know the ins and outs of their most common plans.

The patient may expect it but it's not a reasonable reality. Let's soften the blow of our uncertainty, however. Here are some examples you may use to obtain the information and still send a friendly customer service message.

"Mrs. Smith, we deal with so many insurance companies - I have a good idea about how it may be structured. I'd like to be able to investigate your plan, but it may take an extra call on my part. Are you okay with me calling you back once I find out?"

There's no reason that Mrs. Smith could have to be upset. Now she will likely expect you to know her benefits very well after you offer to check them. That's realistic. But to receive instant benefits for every plan is just too futuristic!

How Much Does My Insurance Cover?

This is the million-dollar question, isn't it? More like a $1000 or $1500 question! When discussing this problematic topic always keep in mind we can never **guarantee** how much is covered. It doesn't matter if you are always correct. The one time that you guarantee coverage, it's going to turn out that the procedure will not be covered.

"How much does my insurance cover?" really means "How much will I have to pay you?" This is the real question. Many of them simply need to plan for the expense of treatment. This is understandable. You'll work with many more patients who are budget-conscious than not.

Rather than saying, "Your maximum for the year is $1,500," (remember we're taking the word maximum out of your vocabulary!) let's try **"Your benefit for the year is $1,500. If we take that from your treatment cost total, then you'll have an out-of-pocket expense of $2,500.**" The patient is asking us to do the math for them. That's the reality and not really unreasonable.

Because many patients won't be able to afford the full cost of treatment without a payment plan, it's important to be flexible by offering third party financing. Extended payments can assist the patient to move forward with treatment but avoids payment plans to the office. I don't recommend you become an in-house bank. The patient could either prepay or make full payment at the time of service. I'm not a fan of extending payment plans for treatment. Too often a patient will delay appointments because they have mentally tied payments to their scheduled appointment. If they are having money issues, it will be easy for them to rationalize canceling their appointment.

However, you know your office's temperature better than I do. If it works for your office, then make sure the follow up on balances is strict and regular. As a general rule, I do not recommend offering payments to your patients other than third-party financing.

Let's go back to communicating how much will be covered. I want to ensure that Mrs. Smith knows I'm familiar with the differences in benefits.

"I'm not sure how familiar you are with your benefits, but we found we're pretty close with our insurance estimates. Keep in mind some plans have clauses which affect how much they cover."

"And Mrs. Smith, I see here you'll need to have an implant placed. I'll need to check if there's a missing tooth clause."

Your clinical team will often be asked these questions. A helpful hygienist or assistant will try to answer this question. This shouldn't surprise anyone – we're customer service oriented and naturally want to help. But I would prefer that the question be kicked up to the insurance coordinator or to the office manager. The person who usually handles insurance conversations should take the patient's concerns and investigate them. Even though the intent is good, sometimes it can be more problematic to give a patient a 'guesstimate' than to direct them to the insurance coordinator.

I am a firm believer that the **team** should know about the most common clauses and how they can affect our estimates. However, when it comes to talking about those clauses and scheduling treatment, I would prefer the insurance coordinator be the one who leads the discussion.

Be sure to enforce that it's a team effort but there is one person on the team for whom this is a primary role. You are acknowledging this team member is the 'expert' in your office.

"If you'd like, I'm going to call in Barb to ask her how she can help you with your benefit questions. If you have any other questions about your treatment, then I'm happy to help you."

Clinical team members are fantastic at talking about clinical issues so I'd like for them to stay in that lane. I also include the doctor in this category. Doctors are notorious for injecting themselves into financial conversations and not always in a good way. , However, some dentists are very capable of taking on this discussion. Make sure this is the case if your doctor discusses finances. Many times, the doctor *thinks* they're good at it but the truth may be that a team member is best suited.

Nervous About Your Co-payment Calculation?

Are you nervous about your co-payment calculation? I speak with new team members who give several reasons why they're not confident in their estimations. These are some of the reasons they give:

- They are working with software that has not been updated with benefits and plan information.
- They're taking over for someone and there is no system in place.

- Fee schedules are not used. This makes it harder for the computer to estimate as it does not take into account adjustments.
- Historical payment amounts are not recorded in the software. Your computer will use these amounts to better estimate the totals.

The unfortunate side of having systems which aren't set up accurately in the beginning is that patients have been taught your co-payments are never accurate. Unfortunately, patients will use this precedent to avoid making payments on their current appointments. You will become more confident as you clean up the system. As the explanation of benefits (EOBs) come back in you'll begin to see how close you're coming to properly estimating totals. Every insurance coordinator has trouble with copayment estimations in the beginning. It's not just you!

When talking with your patients about estimates, let's use language which shows that *you* are in charge of the computer system

"Mrs. Smith - we update the computer when we receive new information about benefit plans. I know it may not have been consistent in the past, but right now, I'm trying my best to get as close as I can."

"We estimate your out-of-pocket for today is $800. I've checked your benefits and made sure the computer is taking them into account. I'm confident this is the best estimate that I can give to you **based on current information**."

You'll notice I bolded that last part. It's because I want you to include the qualifier of 'current information' as it's very important. Your estimate is based on their plan information which – as we know – can be wrong. I urge you to research real-time benefit estimation in your office. Many times, this service can be added into your existing software for a very affordable price. It is worth it so you are not always on the phone. You will be able to collect co-payments faster and you'll be much more confident with your estimations.

Imagine being able to turn your monitor around so the patient can see the insurance company's own estimate. You can also print it out so they have their own record. Being able to say, "Mrs. Smith, look at this. It looks like they have already processed your claim, and you know, it looks like my estimation was right on the nose! Your balance will be $75 today."

What a wonderful feeling when you're able to collect confidently from the patient. That confidence, as I said, will come with time.

Pre-treatment Estimates

Our industry, unfortunately, embraces the pre-treatment estimate. I wish that we did not. You will hear pre-treatment estimates referred to as "predeterminations" or "pre-authorizations. I'd like for those words to be taken out of your vocabulary. Please refer to them as "pre-treatment estimates." When you use the words 'authorization' and 'determinations' you'll hear patients tell you they don't want to proceed because it's not allowed.

Patients tend to request pre-treatment estimates and put off scheduling treatment. Does this sound familiar?

"I know the dentist wants to do five crowns. Can you just send a request to the insurance company?"

I'd love for you to respond in a positive and assumptive tone.

"Sure we can! However, I'd still like to make an appointment for you. I don't want you to fall between the cracks. You know how busy we all get!"

Often the insurance company will send the results to the patient, not the office. You should warn the patient of this possibility. After talking with offices across the country, it's common to hear that pre-treatment estimates only return about 50% of the time. If the insurance coordinator is waiting for a pre-treatment estimate to arrive *before* scheduling the appointment, he or she may be waiting an awfully long time. Let's prepare the patient with:

"We're happy to file it for you, Mrs. Jones. It usually takes several weeks to hear back from the plan. Do me a favor. If the insurance company sends it to you, will you let us know what they have said? Sometimes, they send it to you, and not to us."

"Let's go ahead and schedule your appointment, though. I don't want you to lose track of you!"

When the patient uses a pre-treatment estimate as a delay tactic it allows them to dictate the pace of the insurance conversation. Often it is what they're used to. Let's retrain them by filing the pre-treatment estimate and scheduling the appointment. I have an issue with the dental office letting the patient just waltz out without any follow-up action. Often they'll come back in six months for their preventive appointment and say "what ever happened with that estimate?" and we start all over again. Remember – when they leave through the practice doors you will have a harder time obtaining the appointment.

How to Avoid Insurance-Driven Patient Behavior

It is unfortunate that patients are trained by some dental offices to be insurance-driven. This could also be due to their exposure to the medical side of healthcare. When they visit their medical office for a physical or other appointment, they hear very insurance-focused verbiage. Almost all of the conversation contains limiting terms like "not covered" or "denials."

The dental industry has a different reimbursement model and so our attitude and language has to be different. We have the opportunity to avoid training our patients to be insurance-driven but it will take excellent verbal skills and patience.

When team members make statements such as, "It looks like your plan will cover two of these teeth, but not these teeth over here," and then say, "Well, do you want to go ahead and schedule those two teeth?" What we're implying to the patient is that the insurance company's benefit estimation, or benefit allowance, is what should be dictating their treatment. This is not the case at all. It is our job, as healthcare providers, to present our recommendations on the patient's needs, not on their benefits. We should continue to focus on what conditions are diagnosed and can be treated.

Many services on the dental side are not covered. Insurance companies deem services as elective, aesthetic or cosmetic. These are terms you see often on EOBs of denied procedures. This is also the language patients read on their EOBs.

You'll often find yourself explaining to your patients that the procedure was not elective but was necessary. This conversation is always better to have on the front end when you're talking about recommendations. While you are communicating to the patient the importance of a new crown you can mention that insurance may not provide benefits if they deem it cosmetic in nature.

This prepares the patient and allows them to plan for this instance. It also allows you to reinforce that you will appeal the decision *on their behalf*. Again – we are reinforcing our dedication to customer service. If you wait to explain this after a crown is denied then the patient is already anxious about an unexpected out-of-pocket cost and will likely be upset with you.

Have you heard similar conversation from team members? Keep an ear out for this. You should be doing most of the explanation of aesthetic and non-covered services *before* the treatment is rendered.

If you hear from patients: "Well, they didn't cover it but I know I had to have it done, "then you have done a good job! However, you may hear the opposite reaction of the insurance company doesn't cover it, so I must not have needed it." This reaction means some sort of communication breakdown has happened.

Instead of saying to our patients, "Well, you have got $1,000 maximum, so let's go ahead and just get these three things done," I'd like for you to say, "**The cost of your treatment is going to be $2,000, and that takes into account a $1,000 benefit you receive every year. Your copayment is going to be $1,000. We estimate insurance will cover $1,000, which is your yearly benefit**."

Also offer to work with their plan, but don't let it rule your decisions. Doctors say, "Let's do these two teeth this year, and then next year, we'll do the other two teeth." In my opinion, that is doing a disservice to the patient. We don't even know if the patient can afford to have all of the work done at one time. If the patient can afford to have all of the work done, chances are they will hear you say, "Well, let's do these two teeth," and think, "Okay, I guess the other two teeth aren't that important if the doctor's okay to wait for it."When you phrase it as if the insurance sets the pace then a patient who may be able to afford the complete treatment could believe they *have* to pace it out. Remember, patients will assume that you know their benefits better than they do.

Are You Thinking In Calendar Years?

We can sometimes train patients to think in calendar or benefit years without even realizing it. Listen to your financial and clinical conversations. You may have to retrain your team as this is very common. Almost every office I've worked with has become accustomed to patients wanting to spread their treatment across time. As a result, we anticipate the patient will bring it up and actually begin to do it for them!

Let's train this talk out of your team! There are alternate ways to acknowledge that your patient may need to space out treatment.

- It seems like you want to go slowly. Could you tell me if you have a timeline you're working with?
- Not all of this needs to happen at one time. Are you interested in spacing it out?
- We work with a third party financing company to help you make monthly payments. Would this help?

What you are communicating is that the *patient* should set the pace, not the benefit plan.

I love having a third-party financing company as an option and will include it in planning conversations. These companies make a difference for patients to be able to afford to treatment. Dental work is not inexpensive. Endodontic therapy, crowns and implants are not expenses for which the average consumer usually plans. Even if it's necessary patients will often rationalize forgoing treatment if it is deemed to be unaffordable. Third-party financing makes it affordable for the patient by fitting into their monthly budget. Our patient financing capabilities, whether in-house or by a third party will make a difference for our patients.

Ethics: When Patients Make Special Requests

Oftentimes, patients may ask you to process claims in a questionable manner. This is unfortunate, but we hear this across the country. Patients may ask you to do several actions and they may not realize they're unethical in nature. Here are examples of what you may hear:

- Well, if they're not going to cover that tooth, can't you just bill for this tooth over here?
- The other doctor wrote off my portion – why can't you?
- Bill this on a previous day. I lost my insurance.
- My boyfriend isn't covered. Can you bill my insurance for his work?

Many offices don't realize that all of this is insurance fraud and also is against the American Dental Association's Code of Ethics. If you do feel this is happening in your office, then this becomes a delicate conversation to have with your manager or your dentist. However, it is up to the business owner to ensure this does not happen in your office. Keep in mind that team members may also bear responsibility for fraudulent activity.

One of the first cases I encountered involved a situation in which fillings were not covered because they had been placed previously in another office. The team could not get these fillings covered despite showing that the previous fillings were poorly placed. The office had recommended - and the patient accepted -to replace them with new one and two surface composite fillings. Because of the two-year limitation on restorations all of the fillings were denied.

However, the patient did have coverage for adult sealants. So, guess what the doctor submitted? That's right – the doctor submitted claims for enough adult sealants to come close to the cost of the replacement fillings. We reviewed the records, and it turned out the office had been regularly submitting alternative procedures. They had never been taught that it was wrong and the doctor never checked into the legalities of dental coding and billing. As a result, the office manager was just submitting whatever she wanted to whenever she ran into similar situations. We were able to fix many claims but it was arduous. We wrote letters to insurance companies, returned payments, and contacted patients. It was not an easy process.

Because some offices bill this way, you may encounter patients who expect similar behavior. They also may hear from a friend that the 'office down the street' is writing off co-payments. This method is absolutely unethical and illegal and it's insurance fraud. When a patient asks, "But can't you just submit it this way", these are appropriate comebacks for you use:

- "We would love to help you, Mr. Smith. We want to help you use as much of your benefits as possible, but we have to submit the code that best fits what the doctor did. We don't have a choice on this."
- "Mr. Smith, it's incorrect for us to send it in that way. The doctor's notes match the code we sent in. We have to bill for what is in the doctor's notes, and that particular code that you're asking us to use (or that particular procedure) isn't close to what we did."
- "I know the insurance company told you to do it this way, but we would be committing fraud by sending it in that way." (This verbiage is meant for the limited times a periodontal maintenance is not covered, and insurance companies recommend just sending in a claim using a regular prophylaxis code.)

The last bullet point is alarming because I've been on many calls in which the representatives (from several companies) give this advice. We can't do it this way. We absolutely have to bill for what matches the doctor's notes. The doctor is responsible for letting us know which procedure was performed and as insurance coordinators we ensure that we bill it using the correct code. We have to do what's ethical and right - we would be committing fraud by sending in a claim any other way.

"My Last Doctor Wrote Off My Balance!"

These patients are trained to never make a copayment. How does this happen? Some doctors wrongly advertise that they will not collect patient portions. To them, this is a form of marketing. But we know it's wrong. The doctor more than likely knows it's wrong.

However, the patient doesn't know it's wrong. The patient just thinks they had a good deal for a number of years. Be thoughtful when you hear this from a patient: "My last doctor wrote off the balance. I don't understand why I have to pay you." You should act surprised but be respectful. Remember that patients usually don't realize this is incorrect.

- "That's weird. I know we can't do that here. It's prohibited by our insurance contract and the American Dental Association has guidelines about writing off patient balances."

- "Mrs. Jones, it's prohibited in our contract. We'd be breaking our contract with our insurance companies. , The American Dental Association is pretty clear in their ethical guidelines. The doctor is a member, and she believes that's not how she wants to do business. I'm sorry you had that experience over at another doctor's office, but we can't do the same here."
- "Maybe your last doctor wasn't as familiar with the rules but we have guidelines which we have to go by. I know that if we wrote off your balance, we would be violating the insurance company's and the ADA's guidelines."

When explaining it to the patient, I will point out that I'm following the recommendations of the American Dental Association. According to their guidelines, offices have to bill for what they did and collect for services rendered. Your billing records should match the doctor's notes. Even if a patient continues to argue, you stand firm. Your doctor's license is on the line, and I absolutely don't want anything to happen to your office or your doctor.

Is the patient persistent with their requsts? Try this:

"I'm sorry your plan processed it that way. I'm sorry they didn't allow for benefits. We sent in a lot of documentation so they could make their decision. What I can recommend now is that you pick up the phone and call them, and ask them what more can we do to get this paid?"

I want the patient to become involved in the conversation. If the patient is involved in talking to an insurance company and trying to obtain benefits, there are two sides to this. Number one, they will see just how frustrating it can be to try to obtain benefits. Especially when it's obvious that benefits should have been allowed for certain procedures.

The second point is that when a patient calls they are seen as the policyholder. They have a direct relationship to the employer who is the customer of the insurance company. It is sad to say that as participating providers, we play only a small part in this conversation because we are not the ones who hold a benefit contract with the insurance company. Since the employer and the patient do hold the contract, I like to involve them – especially if I suspect obtaining benefits will be difficult.

"Your Human Resources department could help, Mrs. Smith. I'm happy to give you some information, and maybe they can pick up the phone and call to find out why this claim isn't paid."

Every time a patient involved the HR department the claim has been paid. I show a 100% ratio in getting claims paid once the HR department of a company gets involved. It is amazing how fast this happens when HR or executive of a company complains.

"But I Have Two Plans!"

What about the patient who has two plans (or more!) and doesn't understand why they still have a co-payment? Of all the frustrating conversations we can have, secondary insurance ranks right up at the top of the list. For years, secondary insurance typically meant the patient usually had no out-of-pocket costs. That has changed dramatically. The coverage rates are not the same as they used to be, which is what I want you to convey to the patient.

"For years, Mrs. Smith, having two plans meant no patient portion, but things have changed so much."

"Mrs. Smith – even though you have dual coverage we've found that not everything will be fully covered."

"We're finding, Mrs. Smith, that both plans often don't cover as much as we had hoped. What we can do is try to find out as much as we can before we perform any treatment. If you have the benefit booklet you can bring those in. I'm happy to take a look at it for you."

If a patient's contract has a 'non-duplication of benefits' clause, then we need to be upfront about it. Lack of benefits despite secondary coverage will always surprise your patient.

Simply put this clause means that benefits from the secondary plan will not be paid until the primary's coverage is exhausted.

"Unfortunately, Mrs. Jones, your secondary plan has what we call a non-duplication of benefits clause, and that means it's not going to kick in any benefits until the primary plan has paid out their full benefit."

"Think of it this way, Mrs. Smith. Your secondary plan has non-duplication coverage. It will stay dormant until your first plan runs out."

Hypothetical Situations in Your Office

Your office team has probably run into other situations in which they did not know the right response. In the Appendix you'll find an exercise with which you can work with your team. You'll come up with your own hypothetical situations. I would rather you review these situations *before* they happen than try to regroup afterward.

I'm sure you could point to some recent situations in which you weren't sure that you gave the correct answer. **As a team**, think about some of the situations in which the patients ask questions that throw you for a loop.

I'll give you an example to use as a template and conversation starters. In the meeting with your team, other situations will come up, so be sure to write these down. You don't have to discuss all of them at one time. Discuss a few, or even five at a time so everyone can really pay attention to each other's verbiage. Everybody should be able to go at least once or twice around the circle, around the team table, to discuss how they would have handled it.

Hypothetical Example: Radiographic Refusal

What happens if a patient refuses to have a radiograph taken? How does your office handle patients who don't want to have any taken because they are not covered by insurance? Does the doctor explain that he or she needs the images in order to better diagnose the patient's oral condition? Or do you immediately roll your eyes because we now think Mrs. Smith will be difficult. Be honest!

"Mrs. Smith, Dr. Jones would appreciate being able to take radiographs. He won't be able to see in between your teeth without them. It doesn't look like they'll be covered but we really can't do a thorough evaluation without them. "

Remember that it *is* ultimately the patient's choice. If they're only pushing back because insurance will not cover it then let's talk a bit more with them about it. Radiographic refusal can be a big conversation and can sometimes be emotional. Patients can have medical beliefs as to why they refuse. Other issues can come up such as doctor liability. If a doctor misses a diagnosis for a patient without radiographs it is hard for your malpractice carrier to defend.

Your doctor should look up 'supervised neglect' to make sure he or she is not committing this without meaning to.

The Future of Dental Insurance In Your Office

Dental insurance is becoming more complicated with every year. It used to be a simple contract and both patients and providers who knew what would be covered. Today, offices are dealing with convoluted contracts, hidden networks, and patients who have been told that everything will be covered when, in fact, some procedures are not covered.

The truth is that dental insurance will continue to be more confusing and much trickier to convey to the patient. Patients are not used to looking through their benefits plans. As more exclusionary clauses pop up we'll have to keep our patients informed as to how benefits will be paid.

Our patients will become accustomed to us as their insurance liaison. Comfortable and confident patients will ask us more and more questions about their coverage. Offices that aren't able to step up and offer this help will be left behind because this is the future of dental insurance participation. Offices that are able to show the value of the patients' actual plan, and help them use their benefits in a trustworthy manner will succeed. As business owners and leaders, we are tasked with protecting our practice. We can do this by being alert for insurance changes, consumer trends, and by constantly keeping in touch with our patients. When you and your team are able to establish effective lines of communication with your patients then your bond with your patients can strengthen and grow. Patients will only proceed with needed treatment when they like and trust you. Patients like and trust you when they know you care. Practice your conversations so your patients will realize that they have made the right decision in coming to your office.

May all of your insurance conversations be easy!

Here's How to Have Easy Insurance Conversations That Move Your Patients to Yes!

You have felt the increased presence of dental insurance and how it affects your office. The challenge is the confusion insurance causes among your patients and your staff when all you really want to do is focus on providing good dentistry and quality service.

This is where Odyssey comes in. We help dental offices - just like yours - learn how to have easy insurance conversations that Move Your Patients to Yes!

Step 1: Sign up for and take the online insurance course "Dental Insurance Skills Training." Share the knowledge within your own office. Readers of the book can use "conversations75" for a $75 courtesy.

Step 2: Visit OdysseyMgmt.com to peruse the large library of articles, videos and free webinars.

Step 3: If you would like a dedicated problem-solving session with Teresa, visit her website to reserve a one hour coaching call. We'll gather information from you prior to the call and we'll hit the ground running – but on the phone!

By honing your communication skills, you'll be able to give the right answer to your patients. The more confident your patients feel then the closer you are to Moving Your Patients to Yes!

If you'd like us to help you, send an email to: **Teresa@OdysseyMgmt.com.** Find out why the industry trusts Teresa to keep them informed!

APPENDIX

<u>Fixed Bridge vs. Implant Cost Example</u>

Situation: **Patient opts for a three-unit anterior bridge. Three years later, an obvious bony defect appears.**

Treatment - Round 1:
Total cost of bridge with buildups $ 3,750

Treatment - Round 2:
Cost of corrective treatment three years later:

Bone graft	**$ 1,000**
Implant/abutment/crown	**$ 5,000**
2 crowns (without endo)	**$ 2,200**
Total Cost	**$11,950**

Exercise #1: Avoided and Expensive Procedures

This can be done as a group or individually. For best results, follow this order of brainstorming.

Identify the top 3 procedures that patients seem to dislike the most.

1.
2.
3.

Now what are the results of avoiding those procedures?

Examples of results

- *Physical* results: tooth movement, pain
- *Financial* results: higher cost, lapsed insurance benefits
- *Emotional* results: self-consciousness

Procedure 1

Physical:

Financial:

Emotional:

Procedure 2

Physical:

Financial:

Emotional:

Procedure 3

Physical:

Financial:

Emotional:

Exercise #2: Patient Examples

Every team member should think of a patient in your office who was grateful or emotional when treatment was completed. One patient per team member. Share your experiences and why *you* thought it was so impactful.

Did they smile more?

Did they cry?

What statements did they make? (ex: I never thought I'd smile again)

How have they changed in attitude in recent visits?

Have you asked them for a testimonial?

Exercise #3: Say This, Not That

What terms or phrases can your office say
differently?

Not maximum but benefit
Not cleaning but preventive appointment

Not _____, but
_____

Not _____, but
_____

Not _____, but
_____

Not _____, but
_____

Exercise #4: Hypothetical Situations

Situation:

What is your response?

What should absolutely not be said?

What could change this answer? (new protocols, new materials etc.)

Made in the USA
San Bernardino, CA
14 May 2018